Six-Minute Social Skills 2

Social Detective Skills for Kids with Autism & Asperger's

Janine Toole PhD

Happy Frog Learning

First Printing, 2017

ISBN 978-0-9953208-8-8

Happy Frog Learning

www.HappyFrogLearning.com

About Happy Frog Learning

Happy Frog Learning creates high-quality resources for elementary and high school-aged children with autism and other social/language challenges.

We believe that all children can learn – as long as we provide a learning environment that suits their needs.

www.HappyFrogLearning.com

Social Detective Skills for Kids with Autism & Asperger's

Table of Contents

Introduction: Six-Minute Social Skills

Welcome to the *Six-Minute Social Skills* series. This series is designed for busy parents and professionals who need easy-to-use and effective materials to work with learners who have Autism, Asperger's and similar social skill challenges.

This book, *Social Detective Skills,* provides step-by-step activities that develop strong social radar skills. With the clear and easy-to-use worksheets, your student will learn:

- We all have social expectations about how other people will act.
- We need to be aware of social expectations in order to be socially successful.

Your student will develop the skills to:

- Determine the social expectations of any situation.
- Monitor other people's signals of their expectations.
- Deal with conflicting expectations.
- React appropriately when there is a problem.

These skills are developed incrementally, with lots of practice, allowing your learner to make meaningful progress week by week.

The workbook contains fifty activity pages, organized into two parts. The first four chapters introduce the idea of social expectations - how other people expect us to act – and develops the skills of determining what the social expectations are and if we are meeting them. Each worksheet is preceded by a parent/educator guide containing suggestions for alternate and extension activities.

The final chapter contains 20 worksheets that require your learner to put their new social detective skills to work. Your learner will determine the social expectations in situations as diverse as joining a conversation, dealing with someone who is encouraging bad behavior, and coping appropriately with difficult homework.

Children with ASD need practice at developing their social detective skills. This book is the guide you need to ensure they have the skills to determine, act and react to social expectations in any situation.

Key Ideas Summary

Download a one-page summary of all the Key Ideas introduced in the workbook.

Great for quick reference!

Available for free on our website:

www.HappyFrogLearning.com/Social-Detective-PDF

How to Coach a Six-Minute Session

We want you and your learner to have fun when you coach a six-minute session. So here are some suggestions.

1. Don't worry if you never write in the book!

Filling in a workbook is NOT practicing social skills. What's most important is discussing the ideas and examples that are contained in each worksheet.

So, use the workbook as you need. Use it as a guide for discussion, a guide for oral practice, or as an actual worksheet... whatever helps your student learn something new.

2. Don't be afraid to repeat.

In the six-minute series, we have broken down social detective skills into tiny steps. But even so, your learner will not develop these skills instantly. Don't be afraid to repeat a worksheet until your learner develops confidence.

If you are concerned about boredom, mix your review in with new lessons. In any case, don't move too far ahead if your learner still needs help with earlier skills.

3. Make sure to reciprocate.

A great way to learn is to be the teacher. Once your learner shows progress at a skill, switch the tables so that **you** have to reply. Get your learner to tell you what's wrong with your response.

4. Have a consistent schedule.

Consistency is important if you want to reach a goal. Choose a regular schedule for your six-minute sessions. Get your learner's agreement and stick to it!

We also recommend having a consistent method for delivering each six-minute session. This allows you to move quickly and helps your learner stay focused. Here's a schedule we have found successful.

1. Review the last lesson

Briefly review the Key Idea and activity from the most recent worksheet. Allow the student to see the worksheet as you discuss it.

> *Let's get started. Here's what we did last time. Do you remember what the Key Idea was for that lesson?*
>
> *<wait for student response>*
>
> *Right. And what did this diagram show?*
>
> *<wait for student response>*
>
> *Awesome. Let's see what we do today.*

2. Introduce today's Key Idea

All lessons have a Key Idea. This is a simple concept that is vital for students to know. Once you have introduced a Key Idea, you can reference it when needed during everyday life.

For example, once you have introduced the key idea that everyone in a situation has social expectations, you can remind your learner when he or she considers only his/her own interests.

During a lesson, use a 3-step process to introduce the Key Idea.

1. READ:

   Get your learner to read the key idea, or read it for your student if reading is a challenge.

   > *Here is today's key idea. Can you read it for me?*

2. PARAPHRASE:

   After the student has read the key idea, briefly paraphrase it in a way that is useful for your student's comprehension level.

> *Good reading! So, I guess that is saying that everyone in a situation has their own thoughts about how everyone should behave.*

3. CONNECT:

Talk with your learner about the key idea. Can they think of any examples in their life where the key idea is relevant?

3. Complete & review the worksheet

You can fill in the worksheet by writing or complete the worksheet orally. Either approach is effective.

Provide whatever support is needed to complete the worksheet. Keep in mind that your goal for every worksheet is for your learner to reach the point where they can demonstrate the skill independently.

Once the worksheet is complete, review it together. If your student finds this difficult, you can provide a model. Describe or paraphrase what the student has written/said. Where possible, relate it back to the key idea. For example:

> *I see that you noted that one of your expectations is that if you watch TV, no one will change the channel without asking.*
>
> *That's a reasonable expectation. I have that expectation too.*

4. Extra practice (optional)

Your learner may need extra practice. Most worksheets have suggestions for how to extend the skill development.

5. Revisit the Key Idea

To finish up, draw your learner's attention back to the Key Idea. Ask them to tell you the key idea and then ask your student a question that relates the key idea to the worksheet or to the student's life.

> *Nice job. Now let's look at the Key Idea again. What was our Key Idea?*
>
> *<wait for student response>*
>
> *Yes. We all have expectations about how everyone will behave. Can you think of an expectation I might have if I am talking on the phone?*
>
> *<wait for student response>*
>
> *Fantastic! Yes, my expectation is that I won't be interrupted unless it is really important.*

6. Congratulate your learner & finish

You should provide encouraging feedback throughout the six-minute session. Make sure to also finish up on a positive note. Congratulate your student and identify something they did well during the session.

Have fun!

Chapter 1
What Are
Social Expectations?

Background

In the first chapter, your student learns that everyone has **social expectations**. Social expectations are our expectations about how someone should behave in any type of situation.

Different situations have different social expectations. In a library, there is an expectation that you will be quiet. On a playground, there is a social expectation that you can run around and make noise.

We also have social expectations on a more micro level. For example, we have social expectations for how someone will join a group, for how they will participate in a conversation, etc.

In this chapter, your student learns about social expectations, how they differ from situation to situation, and how we feel if people do not meet our social expectations. At the end of the chapter, your learner will understand that we need to pay attention to social expectations in order to be socially successful.

Coaching Guide: I have thoughts and feelings

Quick Reference:

» Introduce the 'Six-Minute Social Skills' workbook

» Introduce the Key Idea: Read, paraphrase, connect

» Complete & review the worksheet

» Extra practice

» Revisit the Key Idea

» Congratulate your learner & finish

General Notes: The goal of this worksheet is to establish that events and situations cause us to have thoughts and feelings. As we move through different situations during the day, our thoughts and feelings change.

This worksheet is a precursor to the next worksheet where students learn that other people might have different thoughts and feelings about the same situation.

Don't forget, these worksheets can be done orally. There is no need to write the answers – unless you think it would be useful for your student to refer back to later.

Extra Practice: Talk about what happened during today or yesterday and identify what your learner felt/thought at different times.

Your Notes/Extra Ideas:

1.1 I have thoughts and feelings

Key ⭐ Idea

I have thoughts and feelings about

what is happening around me.

Describe your thoughts and feelings in each situation.

Your mom buys you an ice cream.

Your feelings/thoughts _____

_____

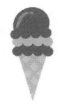

You have some unexpected math homework.

Your feelings/thoughts _____

_____

Your cat has to go to the vet.

Your feelings/thoughts _____

_____

Coaching Guide: Other people have thoughts and feelings

Quick Reference:

>> Review the last worksheet

>> Introduce the Key Idea: Read, paraphrase, connect

>> Complete & review the worksheet

>> Extra practice

>> Revisit the Key Idea

>> Congratulate your learner & finish

General Notes: The purpose of this worksheet is to demonstrate that people may have differing thoughts and feelings about a situation. One person might feel happy. Another might feel sad.

This ability to know that someone else might have feelings that differ from yours is a prerequisite for learning to attend to other people's social signals.

Extra Practice: Talk through the student's day and find situations where the participants might have had differing thoughts and feelings.

After Session: Get your learner to watch out for situations where participants had differing thoughts and feelings. If you are with your student outside of workbook time, point out situations and ask what everyone might be thinking/feeling. You can also do this when you watch movies together or when reading a book.

Your Notes/Extra Ideas:

1.2 Other people have thoughts and feelings

Other people have thoughts and feelings, too.

Their thoughts may be different from mine.

Note down how each person might feel in the following situations.

Maya came first in the spelling test. Her friend Kiera did badly.

Maya _____

SPELL Kiera _____

Ben got a great new camera for his birthday. His brother Alex has always wanted a camera.

Ben_____

Alex _____

It is Ryan's turn to unpack the dishwasher today. His sister did it yesterday.

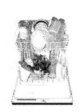

Ryan _____

His sister _____

Coaching Guide: I have social expectations

Quick Reference:

>> Review the last worksheet

>> Introduce the Key Idea: Read, paraphrase, connect

>> Complete & review the worksheet

>> Extra practice

>> Revisit the Key Idea

>> Congratulate your learner & finish

General Notes: In this worksheet, the student learns that they themselves have expectations about how people should behave in different situations. This is a precursor to helping your learner realize that other people have expectations, too.

Once this is established, we can move on to helping our learners realize that we need to pay attention to other people's expectations.

When talking about expectations, be sure to speak about expectations that derive from a situation (social expectations), rather than expectations that are the learner's "wants."

For example, when your learner asks his mom a question, a social expectation might be that his mom answers the question and replies politely. An expectation that you will get ice cream for dinner is a "want", not a social expectation from the situation.

Extra Practice: Step your way through the student's day and talk about what social expectations they have in different situations. Encourage your learner to recognize how their expectations vary from situation to situation.

Your Notes/Extra Ideas:

1.3 I have social expectations

I have expectations about how other people will act.

We call these 'social expectations.'

For each of the situations, put a checkmark next to the behavior you expect.

 I am watching TV in the living room. It's my favorite show.

- It's okay if my brother changes the channel without asking.

- I expect my brother to ask before he changes the channel.

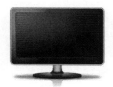 My sister said she would help me with my homework at 4pm.

- I expect that my sister will be home by 4pm.

- I expect that my sister will not be home by 4pm.

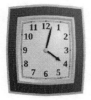 The bell rings for school to start.

- I expect that the teacher will be in the classroom.

- I expect that the classroom will be empty.

Coaching Guide: Often, we have similar social expectations

Quick Reference:

    » Review the last worksheet

    » Introduce the Key Idea: Read, paraphrase, connect

    » Complete & review the worksheet

    » Extra practice

    » Revisit the Key Idea

    » Congratulate your learner & finish

General Notes: In this worksheet, your student learns how most people share the same social expectations for a specific situation. If appropriate, use this information to reassure your learner that they are already an "expert" at knowing many social expectations.

Extra Practice: Talk through the social situations your student experiences during the week and talk about the social expectations. Be sure to talk about general situations like "being in class", "being in the library" as well as more specific situations like "when I see a classmate at the mall" and "joining a conversation."

You might find cases where your learner's social expectations are different from what is needed for the student to be socially successful. These are good opportunities to gently educate your learner about what is more socially expected.

In fact, you are probably already aware of situations where your learner does not have socially successful behavior. They may "topic bomb" (interrupt a conversation with an abrupt change of topic.) They may tune out during conversations. They may interrupt before you are finished answering the question they just asked. Talk through each of these situations with your learner to identify what expectations they currently have and to educate them about what social expectations their conversation partner might have.

These "alignments" of social expectations can be invaluable to your student. So, take as many sessions as you need to bring this awareness to your student.

Your Notes/Extra Ideas:

1.4 Often, we have similar social expectations

Most of the time, all the people in a situation will have the same social expectations.

cial expectation they have.

Everyone should speak quietly.

Teacher supervising playground

It's okay to run around and make noise.

Boy doing homework at the library

Coaching Guide: Sometimes social expectations differ

Quick Reference:

 » Review the last worksheet

 » Introduce the Key Idea: Read, paraphrase, connect

 » Complete & review the worksheet

 » Extra practice

 » Revisit the Key Idea

 » Congratulate your learner & finish

General Notes: The purpose of this worksheet is to ensure your learner understands that his social expectations may differ from those of other people in a situation.

Most of the time, differing social expectations are not a matter of right or wrong. Rather, they indicate the likelihood of the participants being socially successful.

If you completed any of the extra tasks in the last session's worksheets, your learner may already have an awareness of how their own social expectations differ from typical social expectations and how that can reduce the chances of success in social engagements.

If you did not do the extra tasks last time, I encourage you to complete them with your learner either now or when you complete the worksheets for this chapter.

Extra Practice: If you are familiar with your learner, you probably already know the situations where your learner's social expectations differ from those of a neurotypical individual. Now is a great time to talk through some of these situations.

Your Notes/Extra Ideas:

1.5 Sometimes social expectations differ

In some situations,

people might have differing social expectations.

Identify the social expectations for each person.

 Jake is in math class. He is bored so he is drawing on his paper and thinking about camping. The teacher calls out his name in an impatient voice.

Jake's expectations _____

Teacher's expectations _____

How were their expectations different? _____

Lisa's friends Eva and Sue are talking about their homework. While Ella is still speaking, Lisa walks up and says, "Why are you wearing that shirt?"

Eva's expectations _____

Sue's expectations _____

Lisa's expectations _____

How were their expectations different? _____

Coaching Guide: How I feel when social expectations aren't met

Quick Reference:

> » Review the last worksheet

> » Introduce the Key Idea: Read, paraphrase, connect

> » Complete & review the worksheet

> » Extra practice

> » Revisit the Key Idea

> » Congratulate your learner & finish

General Notes: In this worksheet, your learner considers how they feel when their expectations are not met. This is a precursor to later worksheets where they consider how other people feel when their expectations are not met.

Make sure you talk about "social" expectations and not a learner's "wants." See the coaching guide for worksheet 1.3 for further explanation.

Today's worksheet includes three questions for each situation. As a first step, the learner identifies the specific expectations they have. They then identify what the other participants were doing that did not meet the expectations. Finally, they identify how this made them feel. These three steps are important for students to develop their 'social radar' skills.

Extra Practice: Talk through the student's day to see how they would feel in different situations if their expectations were not met.

Your Notes/Extra Ideas:

1.6 How I feel when social expectations aren't met

I get frustrated when other people don't meet

my social expectations.

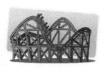 You are talking with a friend about your family hike last weekend. Another friend joins the conversation and immediately starts talking about his plans for going to a theme park next weekend.

What were my expectations?

_____

How did my friend ignore my expectations?

_____

How did that make me feel?

_____

It is my turn to give a talk at school. During my talk, none of the kids look at me. They all stare out the window instead.

What were my expectations?

_____

How did my classmates ignore my expectations?

_____

How did that make me feel?

_____

Coaching Guide: How other people feel when expectations aren't met

Quick Reference:

» Review the last worksheet

» Introduce the Key Idea: Read, paraphrase, connect

» Complete & review the worksheet

» Extra practice

» Revisit the Key Idea

» Congratulate your learner & finish

General Notes: Your learner has probably already experienced people being frustrated with him. This worksheet helps him realize that frustration often happens because social expectations aren't being met.

The three questions in the worksheet give your learner a strategy for figuring out WHY someone is frustrated with them. They can use this strategy in any situation where expectations aren't met.

Extra Practice: Talk about situations you have experienced where you were frustrated by someone ignoring social expectations. Get your learner to answer the three questions about the situation.

Next, get your learner to identify experiences they have had that are relevant. Support your learner in identifying the answers to the three worksheet questions for each situation.

Your Notes/Extra Ideas:

1.7 How other people feel when expectations aren't met

Other people might get frustrated if I ignore their expectations.

Think about social expectations in the following situations.

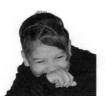 Your teacher is explaining a science topic, but you are whispering and giggling with your friend.

What are the teacher's expectations?

_____

How are you ignoring the teacher's expectations?

_____

How would that make the teacher feel?

_____

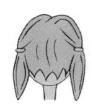 My friend is talking to me, but I turn and walk away before she is finished.

What are your friend's expectations?

_____

How did you ignore your friend's expectations?

_____

How would that make your friend feel?

_____

Coaching Guide: Paying attention to social expectations helps me

Quick Reference:

> » Review the last worksheet

> » Introduce the Key Idea: Read, paraphrase, connect

> » Complete & review the worksheet

> » Extra practice

> » Revisit the Key Idea

> » Congratulate your learner & finish

General Notes: Paying attention to social expectations is hard work, so we need to make sure that your learner is sufficiently motivated to make the effort. They need to **want** to do it.

This worksheet helps the learner realize two important reasons why it is good to pay attention to social expectations. Firstly, we can miss key information if we aren't paying attention to what other people expect. Secondly, others can get frustrated if we ignore their expectations.

If these reasons aren't sufficient for your learner, you will need to think about what will motivate YOUR learner to pay attention to social expectations.

Your Notes/Extra Ideas:

1.8 Paying attention to social expectations helps me

If I ignore social expectations, I can miss important information

and others might get frustrated with me.

 For each of the following social expectations, suggest what could happen if you ignore it.

My mom expects me pay attention to her while she is telling me what to do. If I ignore this,

_____

We should look at the person we are talking to about once per turn. If I ignore this,

_____

If we want to get a drink at the water fountain, we should check if there is a lineup and not just barge to the front. If I ignore this,

_____

We should pay attention to traffic lights. If I ignore this,

_____

When we join a group, we should join in the current topic of conversation. If I ignore this,

_____

Coaching Guide: I should pay attention to social expectations

Quick Reference:

> » Review the last worksheet

> » Introduce the Key Idea: Read, paraphrase, connect

> » Complete & review the worksheet

> » Extra practice

> » Revisit the Key Idea

> » Congratulate your learner & finish

General Notes: This final worksheet summarizes the key idea for the chapter: that we should pay attention to the social expectations for the situation we are in.

Extra Practice: Feel free to add additional social situations that are relevant for your student.

Your Notes/Extra Ideas:

1.9 I should pay attention to social expectations

I should pay attention to the social expectations

for the situation I am in.

 Draw a line from the situation to the social expectation for that situation.

In class	Listen until my friend finishes before I say what I did on the weekend.
Talking with my friend about the weekend	Listen to the teacher.
In the playground	Stay seated at the table and show good table manners.
Eating dinner	Add a comment about soccer.
Joining a friend's conversation about soccer	Run around and have fun.

Chapter 2
How Do We Figure Out Social Expectations?

Background

In the previous chapter, students learned that every situation has social expectations and that it is important to know what they are. In this section, students learn how to figure out what the social expectations are for a situation.

Students practice several strategies for determining the social expectations for a situation. They learn to consider:

- What they know already
- What they see happening
- What people are saying/doing or what they have said/done in the past
- Faces and body language
- And if in doubt, they can ask!

In this chapter, your students learn the detective skills they need to become social experts!

Coaching Guide: I already know a lot

Quick Reference:

> » Review the last worksheet

> » Introduce the Key Idea: Read, paraphrase, connect

> » Complete & review the worksheet

> » Extra practice

> » Revisit the Key Idea

> » Congratulate your learner & finish

General Notes: We don't want our learners to feel overwhelmed by the need to know social expectations in every situation. The purpose of this worksheet is to reassure our learners that they already know a lot about social expectations.

If your learner struggles with the situations presented on the worksheet, make sure to add some additional situations where you know the learner will be successful.

Extra Practice: Talk through the situations your learner encounters at home, at school and in the community. Talk about what the social expectations are in various situations. Commend your learner on how much they already know.

Your Notes/Extra Ideas:

2.1 I already know a lot

I already know social expectations for many situations.

Identify 3 social expectations for each of these situations.

You are at the library to borrow some books.

_____

_____

_____

You are buying candy. There are several people waiting to pay.

_____

_____

_____

You come in to your classroom at the beginning of the day.

_____

_____

_____

Coaching Guide: What are other people doing?

Quick Reference:

> » Review the last worksheet
>
> » Introduce the Key Idea: Read, paraphrase, connect
>
> » Complete & review the worksheet
>
> » Extra practice
>
> » Revisit the Key Idea
>
> » Congratulate your learner & finish

General Notes: The next series of worksheets help your learner hone their observation skills in order to guess what the social expectations are in a new situation. In today's worksheet, your student must pay attention to what other people in the situation are doing.

When your student answers, encourage them to describe how they would think/act from the moment they enter the situation until they are participating actively. They might recognize the general social expectations – for example, they see that they need to join in with the gym class -- but they might miss that they need to do it quietly, without calling out to their friends, etc.

Roleplay can be a fun way to support this learning.

Extra Practice: Talk about other situations that your learner might encounter.

Your Notes/Extra Ideas:

2.2 What are other people doing?

When I don't know the social expectations,

I can look to see what other people are doing.

Identify two social expectations for each of these situations.

You are late for gym class, when you come in, this is what you see.

_____

_____

It is the first day at summer camp. This is what you see when you arrive.

_____

_____

For the first time ever, there is a bunch of people waiting at the bus stop. Usually, it is just you.

_____

_____

Coaching Guide: What are other people saying?

Quick Reference:

> » Review the last worksheet

> » Introduce the Key Idea: Read, paraphrase, connect

> » Complete & review the worksheet

> » Extra practice

> » Revisit the Key Idea

> » Congratulate your learner & finish

General Notes: Other people's words are a big clue that your learner can attend to in order to successfully track social expectations. This can be a challenge for kids with Autism as they may hear the words, but not recognize that there are also social expectations hidden in the words.

Extra Practice: Come up with additional examples from the student's life. Help your learner identify the hidden clues that social expectations are changing. Get your learner to think about whether this is a permanent change or a temporary change.

For example, in the situation where the friend did not like having her name in a song, it is good for learners to realize that they should remember this for next time. That is, the friend gave clues for her ongoing social expectations. She probably didn't just mean to stop now.

Your Notes/Extra Ideas:

2.3 What are other people saying?

When I don't know the social expectations,

I can listen to what people say.

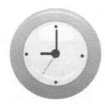 It is Jack's first day at a new school. He walks into the classroom and the teacher says, "Welcome, Jack. Please sit at this desk. I'll introduce you after we've listened to the announcements."

What are 2 social expectations that Jack can figure out?

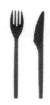 You go into a diner. A waitress says, "Take a seat. I'll be with you in a minute."

What are 2 social expectations you can figure out?

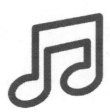 You make up a song with your friend's name in it. She frowns and says, "Stop it."

What social expectations does your friend have right now?

What social expectations might she have tomorrow?

Coaching Guide: What do their faces tell me?

Quick Reference:

> » Review the last worksheet
>
> » Introduce the Key Idea: Read, paraphrase, connect
>
> » Complete & review the worksheet
>
> » Extra practice
>
> » Revisit the Key Idea
>
> » Congratulate your learner & finish

General Notes: In this lesson, your student learns to pay attention to people's faces in order to obtain information about their social expectations. Eye contact is not a strength for many of our learners, so they may miss facial expressions. Looking for social expectations is a good reason for our learners to frequently check in with the people around them.

Extra Practice: Use your knowledge of the student to come up with additional facial expressions and situations for them to practice. Think about how they might engage with siblings, classmates, neighbors, etc.

Your Notes/Extra Ideas:

2.4 What do their faces tell me?

When I don't know the social expectations,

I can look at other people's faces.

Make your best guess about the social expectations.

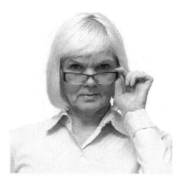

My friend asks me a question in class, I am about to answer him when I see my teacher look at me with this expression.

What social expectations does my teacher have?

_____

_____

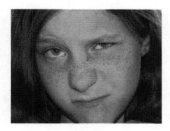

I tell my friend a rude joke. She looks at me with this expression.

What did I just learn about her social expectations?

_____

_____

Coaching Guide: What does their body language tell me?

Quick Reference:

> » Review the last worksheet
>
> » Introduce the Key Idea: Read, Paraphrase, Connect
>
> » Complete & review the worksheet
>
> » Extra practice
>
> » Revisit the Key Idea
>
> » Congratulate your learner & finish

General Notes: Body language can be a powerful communicator of social expectations. In today's lesson, your student learns to check what other people's body positions are communicating.

You might find that your learner needs additional practice with this or previous worksheets as there is a lot of subtlety in how people communicate expectations.

Watching videos can be a great way to practice. At regular intervals, stop the video and talk about what people's faces, bodies and words are communicating about social expectations.

Your Notes/Extra Ideas:

2.5 What does their body language tell me?

When I don't know the social expectations,

I can watch other people's body language.

Answer the following questions.

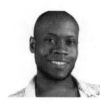

You are whispering with your friend in class. The girl in front of you turns around and looks like this.

What are her social expectations for you at the moment?

_____

_____

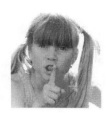

Your dad looks like this when you ask if you can help him.

Why might he look like this?

_____

_____

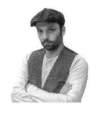

Your dad looks like this when you come in the door from school. Why might he look like this?

_____

_____

Coaching Guide: What do I remember from last time?

Quick Reference:

» Review the last worksheet

» Introduce the Key Idea: Read, Paraphrase, Connect

» Complete & review the worksheet

» Extra practice

» Revisit the Key Idea

» Congratulate your learner & finish

General Notes: Today's worksheet reminds students to think about previous, similar situations to determine what might be expected in the current situation.

For example, if a classmate didn't like hearing their name in a funny song yesterday, your student should remember that information for today. The classmate's feelings are probably the same.

Extra Practice: Where possible add additional examples from the student's own life.

Your Notes/Extra Ideas:

2.6 What do I remember from last time?

When I don't know the social expectations,

I think about last time.

 Yesterday you interrupted your mom on the phone and she was really annoyed. She is on the phone now and you really want to know if she's seen your iPad.

What can you guess about your mom's social expectations right now?

_____

_____

 Last week you made up a fun song that included your friend's name. He didn't like it. You are making up another song today and your friend's name would fit perfectly.

What can you guess about your friend's expectations?

_____

_____

Yesterday your teacher got annoyed when you stared outside while she was talking to you. She will probably talk to you today.

What can you guess about your teacher's social expectations?

_____

_____

Coaching Guide: I can use my judgement

Quick Reference:

» Review the last worksheet

» Introduce the Key Idea: Read, paraphrase, connect

» Complete & review the worksheet

» Extra practice

» Revisit the Key Idea

» Congratulate your learner & finish

General Notes: In today's lesson, students practice using their own judgment about the best thing to do in a social situation. It is important for students to really realize that they already know a lot about social expectations. They just need to actively use the information.

Extra Practice: Give your students some new-to-them situations and ask them to talk-aloud their thought processes for figuring out the social expectations.

Your Notes/Extra Ideas:

2.7 I can use my judgement

When I don't know the social expectations,

I can use my judgement.

Answer the questions about the described situations.

Kian is going to an art gallery for the first time. Choose your best guess for the social expectations at an art gallery.

o Kian should run around.

o Kian should walk around.

o Kian should look at the art.

o Kian should play games on his phone.

Maya is going to her dad's workplace tomorrow for a visit. Draw a line between the workplace and the likely social expectation.

Office building   Speak loudly to be heard over the
                                   machines

Movie set   Speak in a regular voice

Road construction   Be silent when filming is happening

Coaching Guide: I can ask

Quick Reference:

> » Review the last worksheet

> » Introduce the Key Idea: Read, paraphrase, connect

> » Complete & review the worksheet

> » Extra practice

> » Revisit the Key Idea

> » Congratulate your learner & finish

General Notes: Today students learn that they can ask to find out social expectations. This strategy is left until last, because it is not a strategy that students can use in every situation.

Also, it is better for students to use their detective skills to figure things out for themselves, especially when it comes to engagements with peers, who may not be adept at identifying or explaining social expectations.

Do encourage your students to talk to you and/or other trusted adults about any situations they are not sure of, whether it is something that happened, or a situation they anticipate encountering. You (or another trusted adult) should be the person they seek if their detective skills don't give them the information they need.

Extra Practice: Think about situations in your student's life where asking would be the most effective method for gaining information about social expectations.

Your Notes/Extra Ideas:

2.8 I can ask

When I don't know the social expectations, I can ask.

Bryan is about to go to Boy Scouts for the first time. His dad used to be a boy scout and one of the boys in his class goes to Scouts.

Write down 2 questions Bryan could ask his dad and 2 questions he can ask his classmate to find out what the social expectations are at Boy Scouts.

_____

_____

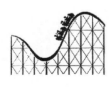

It is lunchtime on Lisa's first day at a new school. Half the students are grabbing their lunches and leaving the classroom. The other half are sitting at their desks. How can Lisa find out what she should be doing?

_____

_____

Jake already has a ticket for the theme park. There is a line in front of the ticket booth and then a line to get in the gate. Jake isn't sure what he should do. How can Jake figure out what he should do?

_____

_____

Chapter 3
How Do I Know
If I Am Meeting
Social Expectations?

Background

In the previous chapter, your student learned to use detective skills to figure out the social expectations for a situation. In this chapter, your student learns to monitor other people's signals to check whether their social expectations are being met.

Students practice several strategies for monitoring social expectations. They learn to consider:

- What people are saying/doing
- How they are saying things
- Faces and body language

By the end of this chapter, your students will have had lots of practice at monitoring how social expectations are being met.

Coaching Guide: I can watch for clues

Quick Reference:

> » Review the last worksheet

> » Introduce the Key Idea: Read, paraphrase, connect

> » Complete & review the worksheet

> » Extra practice

> » Revisit the Key Idea

> » Congratulate your learner & finish

General Notes: In this worksheet, we introduce the idea that people give clues as to whether we are meeting social expectations or not. We can watch for and interpret those clues.

Extra Practice: Roleplay is great for practicing the skills in this chapter. Think about signals you wished your student noticed and roleplay a relevant situation.

Your Notes/Extra Ideas:

3.1 I can watch for clues

To check whether I am meeting social expectations,

I can watch for clues.

You are playing basketball with some friends. The girl with the ball looks directly at you.

What signal is she sending you?

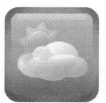

_____

How can you show you are ready?

_____

You are telling a classmate about the video game you played on the weekend. He keeps looking at his phone.

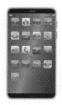

What signal is that person sending you?

_____

What is the best thing for you to do now?

_____

Your social studies group is making a poster. Everyone but you is busy working. The other group members keep looking at you and frowning.

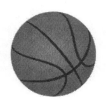

What signals are they sending you?

_____

What is the best thing you can do now?

_____

Coaching Guide: I can listen to what other people say

Quick Reference:

» Review the last worksheet

» Introduce the Key Idea: Read, paraphrase, connect

» Complete & review the worksheet

» Extra practice

» Revisit the Key Idea

» Congratulate your learner & finish

General Notes: The first clue that our learners should pay attention to is what people say. A LOT of information comes verbally. While our students probably understand what people are saying and respond to it appropriately, we also want them to think about what the words mean for social expectations.

Extra Practice: Give your student more situations to consider.

Your Notes/Extra Ideas:

3.2 I can listen to what other people say

To check whether I am meeting social expectations,

I can listen to WHAT other people SAY.

Answer the following questions.

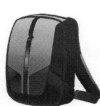

You come into the house, unpack your lunch kit and hang up your backpack. Your mom says, "Great job!"

What social expectations did your mom have?

_____

Did you meet her expectations?

_____

Would you do anything differently next time?

_____

Your shoelace is undone, so you crouch down to retie it. You hear a boy say, "Move out of the way."

What social expectations did the boy have?

_____

Did you meet his expectations?

_____

Would you do anything differently next time?

_____

Coaching Guide: I can listen to how other people say things

Quick Reference:

>> Review the last worksheet

>> Introduce the Key Idea: Read, paraphrase, connect

>> Complete & review the worksheet

>> Extra practice

>> Revisit the Key Idea

>> Congratulate your learner & finish

General Notes: In this lesson, your learner attends to the tone of voice used to communicate.

Your learner may or may not be ready for this lesson. Even if they are not yet great at detecting sarcasm or emotion through words, give the worksheet a try. This will at least introduce them to the idea that information is being communicated through how things are being said, not just the actual words.

Extra Practice: Give additional easier or more challenging examples to suit your learner.

Your Notes/Extra Ideas:

3.3 I can listen to how other people say things

To check whether I am meeting social expectations,

I can listen to HOW other people say things.

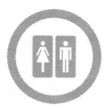 You are at a restaurant and need to go to the bathroom, but you don't know where it is. You ask a man walking by your table if he knows where it is. He gives you an odd look and says, "Do I look like I work here?"

What social expectations did the man have?

_____

Did you meet those expectations?

_____

What would you do differently next time?

_____

You get distracted while putting away your books. Your teacher says to you, "Great job putting your books away."

What social expectations did the teacher have?

_____

Did you meet those expectations?

_____

What would you do differently next time?

_____

Coaching Guide: I can watch faces

Quick Reference:

» Review the last worksheet

» Introduce the Key Idea: Read, paraphrase, connect

» Complete & review the worksheet

» Extra practice

» Revisit the Key Idea

» Congratulate your learner & finish

General Notes: The next clue your learner practices is attending to facial expressions. As noted in the previous chapter, our learners may be weak at using facial expressions as a source of information.

Previously they learned that they can use facial expressions to figure out social expectations. Here your student learns that he can also use facial expressions to determine if he is meeting social expectations. There are lots of reasons why we should occasionally look at the people we are involved with!

Extra Practice: Do a preferred activity together and use your face to convey information about whether your learner is meeting social expectations. You can tally each time he checks your face. You may need to encourage your learner to check in more frequently than his default amount.

Your Notes/Extra Ideas:

3.4 I can watch faces

To check whether I am meeting social expectations,

I can watch other people's faces.

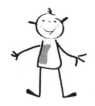

Your mom is preparing dinner, but she looks at you and smiles every now and then as you tell her about the game you played at lunchtime.

What social expectations does your mom have?

_____

Did you meet those expectations?

_____

What would you do differently next time?

_____

Your mom is preparing dinner. She is frowning and flipping through the cookbook pages. You tell her about the game you played, but she doesn't seem to be listening.

What social expectations does your mom have?

_____

Did you meet those expectations?

_____

What would you do differently next time?

_____

Coaching Guide: I can watch body language

Quick Reference:

>> Review the last worksheet

>> Introduce the Key Idea: Read, paraphrase, connect

>> Complete & review the worksheet

>> Extra practice

>> Revisit the Key Idea

>> Congratulate your learner & finish

General Notes: Another one of the strategies that was used to determine social expectations can also be used to check in to see whether we are meeting social expectations. If your learner hasn't noticed that they are using the same skills for two purposes, be sure to let them know!

Extra Practice: Add any additional situations that are relevant to your student's daily life.

Your Notes/Extra Ideas:

3.5 I can watch body language

To check whether I am meeting social expectations,
I can watch other people's body language.

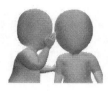
Two boys are whispering to each other in the classroom. As you walk nearby, they turn their bodies away from you and continue whispering. You walk past them and hang up your backpack, then go say hi to your friend.

What social expectations do the boys have?

_____

Did you meet those expectations? _____

What would you do differently next time?

_____

You are first in line at the coffee shop. The coffee shop worker returns to the cash register and punches a few buttons. He doesn't look at you. You start ordering a hot chocolate and the worker frowns while still looking at the cash register.

What social expectations did the worker have?

_____

Did you meet those expectations? _____

What would you do differently next time?

_____

Chapter 4
What To Do When Social Expectations Aren't Met

Background

In previous chapters, your student learned how to determine social expectations and how to check-in to see whether they are meeting other people's social expectations.

In this chapter your student learns what to do if his/her own social expectations are not met. These type of problems occur intentionally and unintentionally through our day.

This chapter helps our students realize that these problems happen and teaches them to match the size of their response to the size of the problem.

Another important issue taught in this chapter is what to do in the case of a mismatch in social expectations. Students must learn to determine which social expectations are most important in a given situation.

An example of a particularly challenging mismatch situation is where an ill-intentioned peer communicates social expectations that lead our student to make poor decisions. The skills taught in this chapter give our students the tools they need to make better decisions in these difficult situations.

Coaching Guide: Ignoring social expectations causes problems

Quick Reference:

> » Review the last worksheet

> » Introduce the Key Idea: Read, paraphrase, connect

> » Complete & review the worksheet

> » Extra practice

> » Revisit the Key Idea

> » Congratulate your learner & finish

General Notes: As a first step in this chapter, we reiterate that ignoring social expectations can cause problems. We want your learner to realize that they themselves can often be the cause of a problem because they ignored a social expectation.

In the next worksheet they learn that other people have these challenges, too, and that sometimes your learner might be affected by it.

Extra Practice: Talk about who was affected by the problems encountered in the worksheet. Talk about what an appropriate reaction from these people might have been... and what would have been an inappropriate reaction.

This will prime your learner nicely for the lessons in the chapter!

Your Notes/Extra Ideas:

4.1 Ignoring social expectations causes problems

Sometimes, ignoring social expectations can cause a problem.

Answer the following questions.

Your teacher is talking at the front of the class. You start telling your friend about your weekend plans to go camping. Your teacher glares at you.

What social expectation did you miss?

_____

How is your teacher feeling right now?

_____

Why is this a problem?

_____

You walk up to two classmates who are already talking and you immediately start talking about your new flip-flops. Your friends glance at each other and roll their eyes.

What social expectation did you miss?

_____

How are your classmates feeling right now?

_____

Why is this a problem?

_____

Coaching Guide: Problems with social expectations happen sometimes

Quick Reference:

» Review the last worksheet

» Introduce the Key Idea: Read, paraphrase, connect

» Complete & review the worksheet

» Extra practice

» Revisit the Key Idea

» Congratulate your learner & finish

General Notes: The purpose of this worksheet is to show your learner that social expectation problems can happen at any time. Sometimes your student will be affected by it. Sometimes they will be the cause of it. Often it is not a big deal.

Extra Practice: Use examples from your student's life where they have been impacted by someone else. You might want to balance the discussion with examples where your student has inadvertently caused a problem by not adhering to social expectations.

Your Notes/Extra Ideas:

4.2 Problems with social expectations happen sometimes

Problems can happen with social expectations, either accidentally or on purpose. That's part of life.

Describe how each person's social expectations are met or not met.

Someone bumps into you in the school hallway. It looks like they didn't notice because they were carrying a big box.

_____

_____

You help your mom carry the groceries in from the car.

_____

_____

Your mom is talking on the phone when you get home, you call out. "Hey, Mom. I had a great day!"

_____

_____

You walk into your brother's room without asking. He glares at you.

_____

_____

Coaching Guide: Problems come in different sizes

Quick Reference:

> » Review the last worksheet

> » Introduce the Key Idea: Read, paraphrase, connect

> » Complete & review the worksheet

> » Extra practice

> » Revisit the Key Idea

> » Congratulate your learner & finish

General Notes: In this worksheet, your student practices classifying problems into small, medium or large.

Don't worry if you can't decide whether a problem is small or medium, or medium or large. The key idea is that some problems are bigger or smaller than others.

Extra Practice: No doubt you will have many relevant examples from the student's own life!

Your Notes/Extra Ideas:

4.3 Problems come in different sizes

All problems, including social problems, come in different sizes.

Draw a line between the problem and its size.

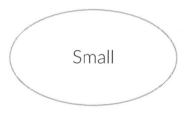

Small

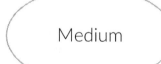

Medium

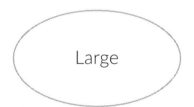

Large

- Your mom went shopping but forgot to get the chips you asked for.

- Someone walking past your desk knocks one of your books onto the floor.

- You tripped in the playground and you think you might have broken your arm. It is swelling and hurting A LOT!

- Your sister calls you a jerk.

- You forgot to bring your math book home and the test is tomorrow.

- You think your dad has cancer.

- You lost a game you REALLY wanted to win.

Coaching Guide: Reactions come in different sizes

Quick Reference:

> » Review the last worksheet

> » Introduce the Key Idea: Read, paraphrase, connect

> » Complete & review the worksheet

> » Extra practice

> » Revisit the Key Idea

> » Congratulate your learner & finish

General Notes: In this worksheet the student learns that reactions come in different sizes.

Like with the previous worksheet, don't get hung up on deciding if something is small or medium, or medium or large. Focus on the fact that reactions can be larger or smaller.

Extra Practice: Draw from your own experience with the student and discuss some of your student's typical reactions.

Your Notes/Extra Ideas:

4.4 Reactions come in different sizes

Our reactions come in different sizes, too.

Draw a line from the reaction to the appropriate box.

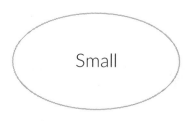

Small

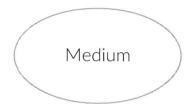

Medium

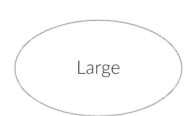

Large

- You shrug your shoulders.

- You call out, "Hey!"

- In a loud voice you say, "I'm not doing that!"

- You say in a calm voice, "Stop it."

- You shove everything off the table.

- You say in a calm voice, "I thought I did finish it."

- You push someone.

- You run out of the room.

- You say, "Okay. I can do that."

Coaching Guide: Reaction size should match problem size

Quick Reference:

> » Review the last worksheet

> » Introduce the Key Idea: Read, paraphrase, connect

> » Complete & review the worksheet

> » Extra practice

> » Revisit the Key Idea

> » Congratulate your learner & finish

General Notes: We can now put the pieces together. Reaction size should match the problem size. So simple. So important. So challenging for many of our students!

Extra Practice: Discuss recent situations where your student has not matched reaction size to problem size.

Your Notes/Extra Ideas:

4.5 Reaction size should match problem size

My reaction to a problem should match the size of the problem.

Draw a line from the reaction to the problem it matches.

- Your mom went shopping but forgot to get the chips you asked for.

- You lost a game you REALLY wanted to win.

- You tripped in the playground and you think you might have broken your arm. It is swelling and hurting A LOT!

- Your sister calls you a jerk.

- You forgot to bring your math book home and the test is tomorrow.

- You think your dad has cancer.

- You ignore her.

- You say, "That's okay. I'll get them tomorrow."

- You tell your mom about the problem and ask her what you can do.

- You say, "Good game." You take a break so you can get over your disappointment.

- You cry and sob because it hurts a lot!

- Before you get too upset, you go talk to your dad.

Coaching Guide: Sometimes expectations conflict

Quick Reference:

» Review the last worksheet

» Introduce the Key Idea: Read, paraphrase, connect

» Complete & review the worksheet

» Extra practice

» Revisit the Key Idea

» Congratulate your learner & finish

General Notes: We now begin talking about situations where social expectations conflict. This often happens cross-culturally. It also happens frequently for our students because they have not absorbed our own culture's 'social norms' in the same way as a similarly-aged neurotypical child.

In fact, this 'different culture' metaphor can work well for students who understand that they have Autism/Asperger's and are happy to discuss differences. You can explain that they need to understand how neurotypical "culture" works, just as they would if they travelled to a foreign country.

Extra Practice: Use examples from the child's own life where social expectation differences have caused conflict.

Your Notes/Extra Ideas:

4.6 Sometimes expectations conflict

Sometimes people's expectations conflict with each other.

Which situations have expectations that conflict with each other? Explain each person's social expectations.

Your friend wants to whisper something to you while the teacher is talking.

You are quiet while you are in the library. You notice the librarians shelving books.

On a field trip to the pool, a classmate tells you to splash a girl when she isn't looking.

Coaching Guide: Deciding which expectations to meet

Quick Reference:

> » Review the last worksheet
>
> » Introduce the Key Idea: Read, paraphrase, connect
>
> » Complete & review the worksheet
>
> » Extra practice
>
> » Revisit the Key Idea
>
> » Congratulate your learner & finish

General Notes: Getting students to recognize a conflict in social expectations is a huge milestone. It won't come easily. However, when they do recognize that there are differing expectations, they need a strategy for how to act.

In this worksheet, we encourage learners to use their own best judgment. Stopping and considering is likely to lead them to a good decision.

Extra Practice: You probably have examples from your student's life where he has made bad choices. Use these as a starting point for discussing differing social expectations and what his best judgement would be now.

Your Notes/Extra Ideas:

4.7 Deciding which expectations to meet

If there is a conflict in expectations,

I use my judgement to decide whose expectations to meet.

Which is the best choice in each of these situations?

A classmate asks to cheat off your homework.

_____

_____

A teammate tells you to trip a player from the other team so you can win.

_____

_____

Your mom has told you not to answer the door when you are home alone. The doorbell rings and you think it might be your friend.

_____

_____

Your mom expects you to wash the dishes after dinner, but you don't feel like doing it.

_____

_____

Chapter 5
Social Detective
Skills in Action

Background

In this final chapter we provide sample situations where your learner can practice the whole range of social expectations skills, from determining social expectations, to checking if the expectations are adhered to, to suggesting modified behavior to avoid or solve problems.

This chapter does not include coaching guides. We are confident you and your student understand the Key Ideas well enough to bring them into play during your discussion.

Each situation has a title. The titles are general rather than specific in order to trigger your ideas for similar situations that are relevant to your student.

For example, the title 'Homework Frustration' could trigger the following ideas for other situations to discuss.

- Other situation(s) where your learner gets frustrated.
- Other situations where your learner reacts like the student in the sample.

There is space at the bottom of each situation page for you to note down other situations you would like to discuss with your learner.

5.1 Hanging out with peers

> *Ben arrives for a playdate at Jim's house. Jim is playing a video game and he doesn't want to stop. Ben stands near Jim, looking bored.*

Answer the following questions about this situation.

What are the social expectations of a playdate?

_____

_____

What are Jim's actions signaling to Ben?

_____

_____

What are Ben's actions signaling about his expectations?

_____

_____

What is the problem?

_____

What are some solutions?

_____

_____

How can this problem be avoided next time?

_____

_____

5.2 Joking in class

> *The teacher asks a question and Jake answers with a joke. One person laughs but a few kids roll their eyes. The teacher glares at Jake.*

Answer the following questions about this situation.

What are the social expectations for answering a question in class?

What do Jake's words and actions signal to the teacher and the students?

For each person mentioned, what are their actions signaling about their expectations?

What is the problem?

What are some solutions?

How can this problem be avoided next time?

5.3 Homework frustration

> *Jeff's mom is helping him with his homework. Jeff still doesn't understand it. He pushes his books away and says, "You're not helping me!"*

Answer the following questions about this situation.

What are the social expectations when someone is helping you?

_____

_____

What are Jeff's words and actions signaling to his mom?

_____

_____

What is the problem?

_____

_____

What are some solutions?

_____

_____

How can this problem be avoided next time?

_____

_____

5.4 Thinking about others around us

> *Erin's mom is waiting outside the classroom to pick up Erin for an appointment. Erin is inside with her class. Erin sees her mom and calls out, "Hi, Mom!"*

Answer the following questions about this situation.

What are the social expectations when you are in class?

_____

_____

What are Erin's words and actions signaling to her classmates and teacher?

_____

_____

What is the problem?

_____

_____

What are some solutions?

_____

_____

How can this problem be avoided next time?

_____

_____

5.5 Noticing when you can help

> *Lori is a teenager. Lori's dad is carrying in bags of groceries from the car. Lori follows him in from the car and says, "I'm hungry. I want something to eat."*
>
> *Lori's dad looks mad and goes back out to the car to get the rest of the groceries.*

Answer the following questions about this situation.

What social expectations does Lori's dad have?

_____

_____

What are Lori's social expectations?

_____

_____

What is the problem?

_____

What are some solutions?

_____

_____

How can this problem be avoided next time?

_____

_____

5.6 Joining a conversation

> *Kasen sees a group of classmates talking and wants to join them. He walks up to them and immediately says, "Hey, what's up?" The girl who was interrupted rolls her eyes and speaks louder.*

Answer the following questions about this situation.

What are Kasen's social expectations as he approaches the group?

_____

_____

What are the speaker's social expectations as Kasen joins the group?

_____

_____

What is the girl conveying with her actions once Kasen joins the group?

_____

_____

What is the problem?

_____

What are some solutions?

_____

_____

How can this problem be avoided next time?

_____

5.7 Noticing lineups

> *Nick is super excited to go on the roller coaster. He runs to the ride gate. A lot of people seem to be near the gate. He hears a few complaining people as he waits for the ride.*

Answer the following questions about this situation.

What are the social expectations in a busy theme park?

_____

_____

What social expectations did Nick miss?

_____

_____

How did the other people convey their frustration?

_____

_____

What is the problem?

_____

What are some solutions?

_____

_____

How can this problem be avoided next time?

_____

_____

5.8 Choosing a topic

> *Yesterday Dave spent a lot of time talking to his friend about his favorite roller coaster. He starts again today, but his friend says, "Not the roller coaster again!"*

Answer the following questions about this situation.

What are the social expectations when talking with a friend?

_____

_____

What are Dave's words signaling to his friend?

_____

_____

What are his friend's words signaling about his expectations?

_____

_____

What is the problem?

_____

What are some solutions?

_____

_____

How can this problem be avoided next time?

_____

_____

5.9 Working in a group

> *Cathy is doing a group project with two classmates. One of them disagrees with everything she suggests. Cathy is starting to feel frustrated, so she is adding, "If it's okay with YOU," to everything she says.*

Answer the following questions about this situation.

What are the social expectations of a group project?

_____

_____

Who is following the social expectations and who is not?

_____

_____

How do you think each person in the group is feeling?

_____

_____

What is the problem?

_____

What are some solutions?

_____

_____

How can this problem be avoided next time?

_____

5.10 Video game manners

Lucas is playing his favorite video game and trying really hard to get to the next level. His dad comes in and says, "Hey, how was your day?"

Answer the following questions about this situation.

What are the social expectations when someone talks to you?

_____

_____

What do you think Lucas feels like saying to his dad?

_____

_____

What should Lucas say to his dad?

_____

_____

What would you do in this situation?

_____

_____

_____

5.11 Accepting the group decision

> *It's recess time and all of Ryan's friends want to play soccer. He doesn't feel like playing soccer today.*

Answer the following questions about this situation.

What are the social expectations when playing with a group of friends?

_____

_____

What is the problem here?

_____

_____

What are some solutions?

_____

_____

Is it okay if Ryan chooses to play by himself?

_____

Describe how Ryan can react if he chooses to play with friends and if he chooses to do something else.

_____

_____

How do you expect his friends to react in each situation?

_____

5.12 Watch out for expectations that might get you into trouble

> *Jason thinks that Keira likes him. Max tells Jason that he should go and hug her.*

Answer the following questions about this situation.

What are Max's social expectations for Jason?

_____

_____

What are the social expectations around hugging?

_____

_____

Are there any conflicts in social expectations in this situation?

_____

_____

What is the problem?

_____

_____

What are some solutions?

_____

_____

How can this problem be avoided next time?

_____

_____

5.13 What's okay to touch

Lisa's aunt puts her phone on the table. Lisa is curious about it so she picks it up and starts playing with it. Her aunt grabs it from her and says, "What are you doing?"

Answer the following questions about this situation.

What are the social expectations when it comes to other people's possessions?

_____

_____

What are the aunt's words and actions signaling about her expectations?

_____

_____

What is the problem?

_____

_____

What are some solutions?

_____

_____

How can this problem be avoided next time?

_____

_____

5.14 Avoid interrupting

> *Two teachers are talking in the hallway. A student named Raya walks up and says, "When is the math homework due?"*
> *Both teachers frown at Raya.*

Answer the following questions about this situation.

What are the social expectations when two people are talking?

_____

_____

What were Raya's social expectations when she approached the teachers?

_____

_____

Are there any conflicts in social expectations in this situation?

_____

_____

What is the problem?

_____

What are some solutions?

_____

_____

How can this problem be avoided next time?

_____

_____

5.15 Keep your reaction to the right size

Kian asks his teacher if he can go to the washroom. She says he has to wait until school finishes in 3 minutes. Kian raises his voice and says, "I have to go NOW!"

What are the social expectations when you are in class?

What are the social expectations of talking to a teacher?

Are there any conflicts in social expectations in this situation?

What is the problem?

What are some solutions?

How could Kian have acted if he did urgently need to go to the washroom now?

How can this problem be avoided next time?

5.16 Don't make fun with names

> *A classmate named Elijah walks into the classroom. Max sings a fun song with Elijah's name in it. Elijah scowls at Max.*

Answer the following questions about this situation.

What are the social expectations around using people's names?

_____

_____

What are Elijah's actions signaling about his expectations?

_____

_____

What is the problem?

_____

_____

What are some solutions?

_____

_____

How can this problem be avoided next time?

_____

_____

5.17 Show you are interested

> *While my friend tells me about her visit with her grandma, I hum a little song quietly.*

Answer the following questions about this situation.

What are the social expectations when you are having a conversation?

_____

_____

What are my words and actions signaling to my friend?

_____

_____

What is the problem?

_____

_____

What are some solutions?

_____

_____

How can this problem be avoided next time?

_____

_____

5.18 Stay on your friend's topic

> *Ben's friend Grace tells him she went camping on the weekend.*
>
> *Ben says, "Good. What do you have for lunch today?"*

Answer the following questions about this situation.

What are the social expectations when you are having a conversation?

_____

_____

What are Ben's words and actions signaling to Grace?

_____

_____

What is the problem?

_____

_____

What are some solutions?

_____

_____

How can this problem be avoided next time?

_____

_____

5.19 Don't gang up on anyone

> *Gary and a friend are playing at Gary's place. Gary's little brother John is being annoying so they hide from him and laugh when they hear him calling.*

Answer the following questions about this situation.

What are the social expectations when there are people you want to play with and people you don't want to play with?

_____

_____

What are Gary's words and actions signaling to his brother?

_____

_____

What are John's words and actions signaling about his expectations?

_____

_____

What is the problem?

_____

What are some solutions?

_____

_____

How can this problem be avoided next time?

_____

5.20 Politeness, even when you disagree

> *Maya's neighbor tells Maya that she should do better in school.*
>
> *Maya says, "You're not the boss of me."*

Answer the following questions about this situation.

What are the social expectations when you are having a conversation?

_____

_____

What are Maya's words signaling to her neighbor?

_____

_____

What is the problem?

_____

_____

What are some solutions?

_____

_____

How can this problem be avoided next time?

_____

_____

What Next?

Check out the other books in our Six-Minute Social Skills series!

Available on Amazon or at www.HappyFrogPress.com

Key Ideas Summary

Download a one-page summary of all the Key Ideas introduced in the workbook.

Great for quick reference!

Available for free on our website:

www.HappyFrogLearning.com/Social-Detective-PDF

Need More Resources?

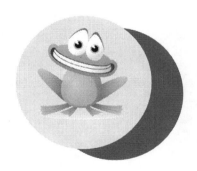

www.HappyFrogLearning.com

Happy Frog Learning creates quality resources for elementary and high-school children with autism and other social/language challenges.

Our award-winning apps, workbooks and curriculums target reading comprehension, social skills and writing.

CERTIFICATE
OF
ACHIEVEMENT

THIS CERTIFICATE IS AWARDED TO

_____

IN RECOGNITION OF

_____

_____   _____

DATE   **SIGNATURE**